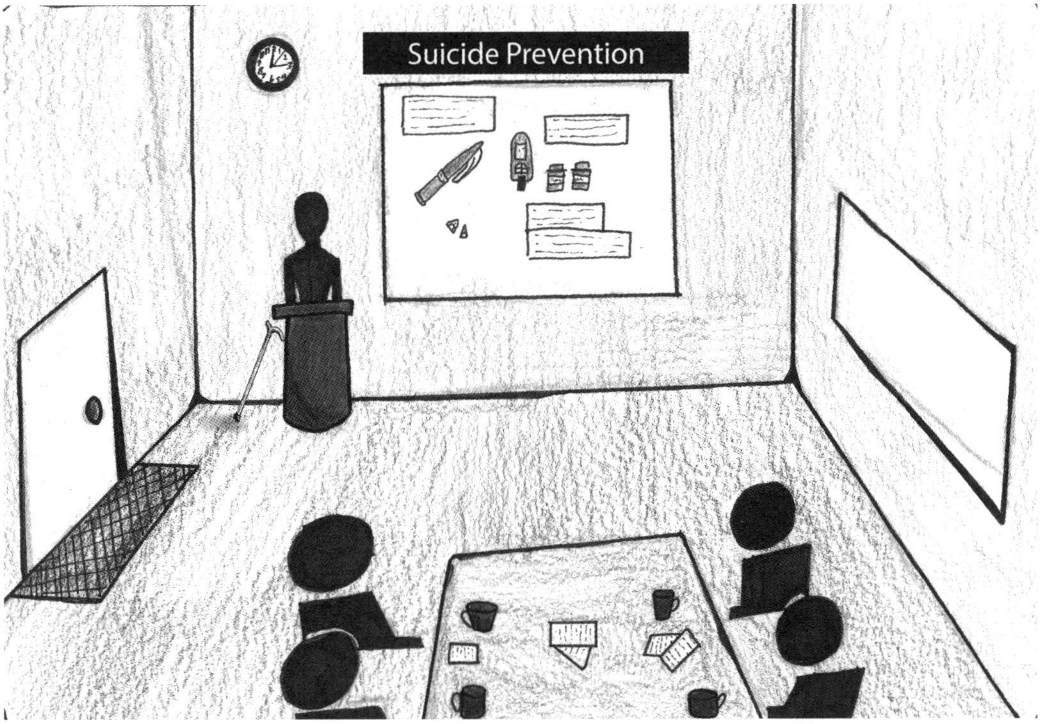

Jack Otter odibaajimowin imaa Waaswaanibiing
The Story of Jack Otter of Waswanipi

Told by Jack Otter
Written by Ruth DyckFehderau
Translated into Ojibwe by Patricia M. Ningewance

ᒋᔦᐲᒥᑎᓲᐅᓐ ᐊᓈᓈᑭᒋᐦᒑᑭᓈᒡ
CONSEIL CRI DE LA SANTÉ ET DES SERVICES SOCIAUX DE LA BAIE JAMES
CREE BOARD OF HEALTH AND SOCIAL SERVICES OF JAMES BAY

Funding for this publication was provided in part by Health Canada. The opinions expressed in this publication are those of the storyteller and do not necessarily reflect the official views of Health Canada or of the Cree Board of Health and Social Services of James Bay.

Some names and details in this book may have been changed for the purpose of protecting identities. Any similarities between these changed names or details and real persons, living or dead, is not intended.

First printing, 2020. Printed and bound in Canada by Houghton Boston Printers, Saskatoon, Saskatchewan. Distributed by Wilfrid Laurier University Press / wlupress.wlu.ca

Set in Verdana font, chosen for its readability. Printed on paper that is Forest Stewardship Council-certified with post-consumer recycled fibres, and that is acid- and chlorine-free.

Cover design by Nicole Ritzer, based on an original design by Cameron Mosimann. Photograph of Mistissini burnt forest (reversed) taken by David DyckFehderau. Title page illustration by Jared Linton of Mikw Chiyâm Arts Concentration Program, Voyageur Memorial High School, Mistissini, QC.

Published by Cree Board of Health and Social Services of James Bay
Contact: Paul Linton, 168 Main St, Mistissini, QC, Canada, G0W 1C0 / (418) 923-3355
creehealth.org / sweetbloods.org

Library and Archives Canada Cataloguing in Publication

Title: Jack Otter odibaajimowin imaa Waaswaanibiing = The Story of Jack Otter of Waswanipi / written, Ruth DyckFehderau ; told, Jack Otter ; translated into Ojibwe, Patricia M. Ningewance.

Other titles: Story of Jack Otter of Waswanipi

Names: DyckFehderau, Ruth, author. | Container of (work): DyckFehderau, Ruth. Story of Jack Otter of Waswanipi. | Container of (expression): DyckFehderau, Ruth. Story of Jack Otter of Waswanipi. Ojibwa. | Cree Board of Health and Social Services of James Bay, publisher.

Description: "A Story from The Sweet Bloods of Eeyou Istchee: Stories of Diabetes and the James Bay Cree." | Text in Ojibwa and English.

Identifiers: Canadiana 20200218549 | ISBN 9780973054262 (softcover)

Subjects: LCSH: Otter, Jack (Of Waswanipi)—Health. | LCSH: Diabetics—Waswanipi (First Nation)—Biography. | LCGFT: Biographies.

Classification: LCC RC660 .D92 2020 | DDC 362.1964/620092—dc23

Imaa oodenaang Waswaanipii, Kwebek, ayaa bezhig inini Jack izhinikaazo. Giishpin waabamig bagizoyin imaa Waswaanipiiwi-ziibiing gi-ga-waabanda'ig aaniindi imaa gaa-izhi-waagijiwang ziibi gaa-gii-izhi-jekibiinang okaadan, gichi-giigooy shark gaa-inind o-gii-giishkandaan bezhig okaad.

Gaawiin wiin iwe owe dibaajimowin.

Gii-oshkiniigiinsiwid Jack Otter, bagwadakamig gii-izhidaawa' oniigi'igoo'. Wiin dash wiin gii-gikino'amaagozi. Gii-biibooninig odoozisan o-gii-wiijidaamaan imaa Waswaanipiing. Gii-minwaadizi. Weweni o-gii-ganawenimaan odoozhiman awe ikwe. O-gii-minwendaan dash bagwadakamig gii-dazhiiked Jack. Ezhi-gashkitood ako gii-izhaa noopimiing. Niibiwa oshkiniigiinsag o-gashkitoonaawaa ji-gii'osewaad baashkizigan e-aabajitoowaad. Gewiin Jack. Odeden dash gaye o-gii-gikino'amaagoobaniin ji-aabaji'aad mitigwaabiin gaye ji-aabajitood basitebijigan. Aabiding gii-bimi-ayaagoban wemitigoozhi imaa Iiyoo-ischiing, o-gii-mazinaakizwaan Jaakwan e-basitebijigenid. Mazina'iganing dash gii-ate iwe mazinaakizon.

Gii-oshkiniigiinsiwid Jack, gii-maajii-ziizibaakwadwaapine. Mashkikiiwikwen o-gii-wiindamaagoon ji-amwaad mashkikiinsan giishpin zaabamanji'osig. Mazina'iganens gaye o-gii-miinigoon

In the town of Waswanipi, Québec, lives a one-legged man named Jack. If he sees you swimming in the Waswanipi River, he will show you the river bend where he once submerged his legs and a school of hungry river sharks came along and nibbled one right off.

This is not that story.

When Jack Otter was a teenager, his parents lived in the bush. He had to go to school, though, and during the school months he stayed with his aunt in Waswanipi. She was kind and provided a safe home for him in the times he couldn't be with his parents. Still, living on the land was his true way of life and he went out to the bush as often as he could. Like most young Cree in the '80s, Jack could hunt with a gun, but his father had taught him the traditional ways of hunting with bow and arrow or slingshot. An anthropologist came through Eeyou Istchee once and took a photograph of the boy Jack and he published it in a book. In wide-legged stance, Jack is pulling back the band of a slingshot, aiming at some kind of small game.

When Jack was a teenager, he learned that he had diabetes. The nurse said it just meant he should eat a candy if he felt weak and gave him a pamphlet. People with diabetes should eat better,

1

ji-agindang. Gaa-ziizibaakodwaapinewaad nawach babenak daa-inanjigewag gii-ikidoomagan iwe mazina'iganens, gaawiin dash wiin gii-ikidoomaganzinoon wegonen ge-miijiwaapan. Gaawiin igo aapiji o-gii-nisidotanziin ekidoomaganinig iweni mazina'igan Jack. Gaawiin aapiji igi mashkikiiwikweg gaye mashkikiiwininiwag o-gii-gichi-inendanziinaawaa iwe inaapinewin. Gaawiin gii-wiisagendanzii. Gii-minomanji'o. Ngoding ako gaawiin zii-zaabamanji'osii gemaa gii-gichi-minikwe nibi giiyaabi dash e-wii-minikwed. Gii-nitaa-minikwe zhingobiiwaabo owiijiiwaagana' e-wiijiiwaad. Gii-jiigikamigizi aaniish naa gii-midaaso-shi-nishwaaso-biboone.

Gii-giizhininiiwid Jack gii-anokii, noopimiing enaagajitood bagwadakamig. Ngoding ako gii-anokiid noopimiing, gaawiin ako zaabamaji'osii. Odamwaan ako mashkikiinsan, gaawiin dash ginwesh minomanji'osii, aazha miinawaa ko nibaase odoodaabaanensing epiich-zaabamanji'osig. Amii ngwana iweni omiskwiim gaawiin de-ayaamagazinoon ziiizibaakwad wenji-inamanji'od. Gii-maajii-minikwe gaye Jack. Nawach aanjiike gii-maanzhi-ayaani omiskwiim. Ngoding ako gii-waniike, e-gashkitoosig ji-goshkozid ndawaa ko aakoziiwigamigong gii-izhiwinaa.

it said, but it didn't explain what "eating better" meant. In fact, it didn't really say anything that made sense to Jack. Obviously, whatever diabetes was, the doctors and nurses weren't taking it seriously so it couldn't be too bad. He wasn't in pain and most of the time he felt fine. It could sometimes be inconvenient – he would run out of energy, or drink jugs of water without quenching his thirst – but it didn't interfere with more important things in life. Like parties on the weekends. Or a quick high now and then. Or the pleasure of a cold beer (or five, or ten) after school with his friends. In his whole life, he would be 18 years old only once. It was important to make the most of it, to have as much fun as he possibly could.

Jack became a conservation officer and, on the side, he studied further to be a game warden. Sometimes at work he suddenly felt much too weak to do the work forestry guys do, and he didn't always remember to carry a piece of candy. When he did remember, the candy worked only a short time; after a half hour or so, he would be right back where he started (asleep in the truck). He didn't know it, but his sudden weakness came from erratic blood sugar levels caused by diabetes. Frustrated and wanting to escape the cycle but not knowing how, Jack began to drink more than before. His sugar levels became even more erratic, and once a month or so he collapsed into a diabetic or hypoglycemic coma and someone would have to take him to the hospital.

Biinish o-gii-nisidawinaagoo' gaa-anokiinid imaa aakoziiwigamigong. "Gi-zaagitoonaadog omaa bizhishig gii-biizhaayin," odigoo' ebaapizhimigod. "Gi-minopidaanaadog owe miijim, gemaa gi-minonawaak ogo mashkikiiwikweg."

The people at the hospital all recognized him. "You must really love it here, Jack," they would joke. "It must be our tasty hospital food. Or comfortable beds. Or maybe it's our cute nurses."

Gii-miinaa dash mashkikiwa', miinawaa dash ako ando-anokii.

A few days later, with pills or insulin in hand, he'd be back at work again.

Igi gaa-anokiiwaad bagwadakamig nitaa-baazigosewag gii-danakamigiziwaad noopimiing, zagaakwaang. Wiiba ko wiinawaa godak ininiwag giigewag giishpin miskwiiwiwaad ozidiwaang okaadiwaang. Wiin dash wiin Jack ginwesh ako jibwaa-giiged. Ngoding bangii gii-baazigosed amii ezhi-maajii-miniiwid. Gii-onaagoshininig ako baagininjii gaye baagizide. Gaawiin gaye aapiji na'aabisii. Aabiding gii-maajizhwaa oshkiinzhigong ozaam e-biigiziwinang. Niibiwa gegoon maanzhi-ayaa. Namanch ge-gii-izhichiged, inendam.

All the guys at work knew that forestry jobs involve getting scratched up by branches and insects. No one really complained about it. Jack began to notice that his scratches took weeks to heal but his friends' scratches healed in a few days as usual. Shallow scrapes that barely showed up on Jack's skin began to infect. At the end of the day, when he came home from work, his hands and feet were swollen. He was having a hard time seeing clearly too. Eventually, his vision got so cloudy that he needed laser eye surgery just to be able to do his work. So many health problems. Sure, they all seemed minor, but they were getting to be annoying. If only there were something he could do.

2004 dash gii-izhisenig, gii-anokii imaa Radisoning aki enaagajitood. O-gii-wiijiiwaan bezhig wiijiiwaaganan

In 2004, Jack was working as a conservation officer in Radisson. He and a friend attended a golf benefit in Val D'Or imaa Val D'Or gegoon e-inakamiganinig agwajiing. Golf gaa-izhinikaadeg odaminowag. O-giiwewinaawaabaniin dash ini odaabaanensan wenji-waabandamowaad gegoon e-atenig miikanaang gaa-apizowaad. Wewiib aana-gii-oshkibizo awe Jack owiijiiwaaganan ozaam dash enigok. Gii-aaboojisewag, Jack dash okaad gii-badagoshkoodeni.

Aana-zaagijibani'o Jack owiijiiwaaganan e-mayaawiwebinaad ini odaabaanensan. Gaawiin dash o-gii-gashkitoosiin Jack ji-niibawid. Gii-bookogaadeshin iinzan. Amos Aakoziiwigamigong o-gii-izhiwinigoon Jack owiijiiwaaganan. Gii-na'iganesijigaadeni okaad, gii-asiniikandaadeni gaye, gaye mashkikiwa' gii-miinaa ji-wiisagendanzig aapiji. Gii-giiwe dash Waswaanapiing ji-giiged okaading.

Aapiji gii-gichi-wiisagendam imaa okaading gaa-gii-izhi-bookoganeshing. Ngoding ako gii-dibikaninig gaawiin ogashkitoosiin ji-nibaad. Wii-zhiishigagowe, gaye gabegiizhig gaawiin zaabimanji'osii, niningishkaa gaye. Amii iwe enaak e-bookoganeshing, amii maawiin enendaagwanogwen gii-inendam. Zhaagooch dash mashkikiiwigamigong gii-izhaa, e-andooshkang mashkiki ji-onji-minomanji'od. O-ganawaabamigoon mashkikiiwininiwan. Gaawiin giiyaabi daa-apiichi-wiisagendanzii e-gii-bookoganeshing odinenimigoon.

and were returning the golf cart to its parking place when they saw something just ahead on the road. Jack's friend swung the driver's wheel to avoid it, and the cart swerved – a little too much. It flipped right over and landed partly on Jack's upside-down leg.

Jack's friend got out and pushed the cart upright again and helped Jack to his feet. But Jack couldn't stand on his leg. It had broken in the accident. His friend took him to the Amos hospital where the doctor set the leg and casted it, gave him something for pain, and Jack went home to Waswanipi to heal.

The leg hurt. It really hurt. Sometimes Jack would wake in the night wanting to vomit, and all day long he felt weak and shaky. It was his first broken bone; probably all healing broken bones felt like this. Still, Jack went to the clinic and asked for a pill to control the nausea and weakness while his leg healed. The doctor eyed him strangely. The pain should have subsided long ago, the doctor said, and nausea and weakness were not actually symptoms of broken bones. He reached for his small electric saw, sawed off the cast, and lifted it away.

Gaa-izhi-baakizhang iweni gaa-gii-izhi-asiniikandaazonid, e-baakinang.

Wiinge ngwana miniiwigaade Jack. Bishagizhagayeshkaa, gaye baagise, wiinge waasikwaani ozhagay gaye miskozhagaye gaye bangii ozhaawashkozhagaye. Gichi-miniiwi Jack, bichiboowinini dash okaad, amii gaa-onji-wii-zhashigagowed. Gaawiin o-gii-gikendanziin Jack iwe ziizibaakwadwaapinewin naa gaa-onji-giigesig. Gaawiin anokiimagazinini iwe obiskwad ji-gashkitood ji-giiged. O-gii-beki'igoon mashkikiiwininiwan gaye mashkikiwan e-gii-miinigod ji-gagwe-giiged...

...Waasa wedi aakoziiwigamigong Montreal gii-izhi-goshkozi Jack. Gaa-bimisemagak iinzan gii-aabajichigaadeni ji-izhiwinind. Gaawiin gii-mikawisii iwe gii-izhiwinind. Iweni gaa-bichiboowininig okaad gaa-gii-onji-gashkitoosig gwayak ji-inendang.

Apii gii-goshkozid Jack, o-gii-wiindamaagoon ini mashkikiiwininiwan imaa Montreal gaa-ayaanid gaawiin iinzan gwayak gii-ziidosijigaadesinini okaad gii-bookogaadeshingiban. Aana-gagwe-giigemagan iinzan iwe okan, gaawiin dash gii-gwayakisinzinoon, gaye dash oziizibaakwadwaapinewin gaa-gii-onji-gashkitoosig ji-giiged. Miinawaa o-gii-ziidosidoonaawaa iwe okan, miinawaa

Jack's leg was obviously infected. The skin was peeling and the area around the break was swollen and shiny and red and purple and green. The infection had filled Jack with toxins and was making him nauseous. Jack didn't know it, but his diabetes was preventing healing; his pancreas was too burned out to create the hormones that help the body heal. The doctor cleaned up the skin, gave Jack antibiotics for the infection...

...And Jack woke up hundreds of kilometres away in the hospital in Montréal. He had been airlifted there. He remembered none of it. The infection in his broken leg had poisoned his blood so badly that it had even affected his ability to think.

Once Jack was fully awake and alert again, the Montréal doctor told him that, way back on the day of the accident, the doctor in Amos hadn't set the broken leg properly. The bone had been trying to heal for months now, but, because of the improper bone setting and because of his diabetes, it had made no headway at all and was as broken and infected as ever. They re-set the bone then and tried to ji-gagwe-giigemagak. O-gii-atoonaawaan onagizheyaabiinsan biinjiya'ii okaading gaa-izhi-wiiyaasiwid, ji-inaazhigawig iwe mini, ji-zaagidaazhigawig ji-ayaasinog bichibowin imaa. Nasine o-gii-aanjiiginaanaawaan agobizoniiginoon, bizhishig e-naagajitoowaad iweni.

Aapiji o-gii-zhiingendaan e-goskwaawaadabid Jack. Omaa Montreal aakoziiwigamigong gii-baatiinowag godag omashkiigoog. Gii-babaamaagoweba'odizo imaa odesabiwining emawadisaad. Aaninda gaawiin gii-zhaaganaashiimosiiwag gaye gaawiin gii-baakwaa'ishiimosiiwag. Aapiji o-gii-jiikendaanaawaa awiyan e-omashkiigoomonotaagowaad. Wiiba go o-gii-waabandaanaawaa igi mashkikiiwininiwag e-omashkiigoomonid. Amii gaa-inaabaji'aawaad ji-aanakanootamaagenid gii-ayaanid awiyan gaa-michi-omashkiigoomonid. Moozhag ako gii-babaapiwag igi omashkiigoog, Jack e-gaganoonaad e-baapiwaad igi. Gii-minwendam gegoon e-inaabadizid miinawaa. (Namanch gaa-izhichigewaagwen igi omashkiigoog awiyan gii-ayaasinig imaa ji-aanakanootamaagowaad?)

Gegapii gii-giiwe wedi Waswaanapiing Jack e-gii-izhaad imaa mashkikiiwigamigong ji-ando-waabamind. Aabiding e-bimaakoweba'odizod imaa biindig,

give the leg another chance to heal. They inserted – right into the flesh – narrow tubes that collected the extra pus and fluids and carried them out of the leg so they couldn't trap toxins inside. They changed the bandages often, always checking the healing flesh very carefully.

Jack hated sitting still. In this Montréal hospital were many other Cree people, so he passed the time by wheeling himself around and visiting them. Some of the older ones didn't speak English or French and were so grateful to have someone there to talk with in their own language. It didn't take long at all for the doctors and nurses to realize what Jack could do, and soon they came for him whenever they had to do a procedure on a Cree person who couldn't speak their languages. Jack wheeled himself into the room and translated for the doctors and the Cree patients. All the while, he visited and joked with the Cree folks in their own language to take their minds off of all of these strange procedures and of the scary place they were in. It felt so good to be useful again. (But what did all the elderly Cree do when no one was there to translate for them? Did they just suffer in fear and silence?)

Eventually, Jack went back home to Waswanipi, where he dutifully stopped by the clinic regularly for check-ups. One day, making his way on crutches around gii-ozhaashishin edipaabaawesagaanig. Apane gii-gawise.

Amii apan!

Aapiji gichi-wiisagishin imaa godag okaading gaawiin gaa-gii-izhi-bookogaadeshinzigiban. Amii gii-baasigidweshing. Amii apane ogidigoon. Ishe hay.

Zhemaak mashkikiiwininiwa' Shibogmoong o-gii-izhinizha'ogoo'. Amii dash imaa bezhig bakaan mashkikiiwinini o-gii-ago'aan biiwaabik imaa ogidigong ji-ziidopizonid ogidigoon gaa-gii-izhi-baasisimaad, weweni ji-giiged. Amii dash miinawaa gaa-izhi-gagwejii'ind ji-zoongigidigwed. Ngoji go gegaa ango-giizis gii-izhisenig gii-maajii-giige imaa ogidigong.

Godag dash iwe okaad gaa-gii-bookosidoopan gii-bichishing odaabaanensing giiyaabi wiisagendam. Aabiding dash e-onaagoshininig gii-ishkwaa-wiisiniwaad, Jack noojigo maajii-ikido egaagiigidod. Omaamaan oganawaabamigoon. Zhemaak aakoziiwidaabaanan o-gii-andomaan e-gikendang gegoon e-izhiiyaanid ogozisan. Igi mashkikiiwininiwag imaa gaa-ayaawaad mashkikiiwigamigong Montreal zhemaak o-gii-izhinizhawaawaan ji-inaashinid.

the halls, he hit a patch of wet floor and wiped right out.

CRACK!

A sharp familiar pain shot through his good leg. He had busted his knee. The good one. Of all the dumb luck.

The clinic doctors sent him in an ambulance to the hospital in Chibougamau where a surgeon drilled a plate into the knee to stabilize it so Jack could heal properly. Then came weeks of exercise and rehabilitation, but soon enough the good leg with the busted knee healed.

The other leg, the one broken in the car accident, continued to hurt. One evening, after dinner, Jack began speaking gibberish to his Mom. She looked at him closely, right in the eye – and then called the ambulance. The doctors at the clinic had Jack airlifted to Montréal.

Gaawiin gii-giigesinini okaad Jack. Aazha ningodwaaso-giizis odaana-dazhiikaagoo' mashkikiiwininiwa' gaawiin dash giigesii gaa-izhi-miniiwigaaded. Gaawiin ayaasinini wiiyaas okaading bangii, bizaanigo gi-waabandaan okan. Aapiji dash wiisagendam.

"Ndawaa nin-ga-manizhaamin gikaad," odigoon mashkikiiwininiwan. Ogikendaan Jack iwe ndawaach ji-izhisenig.

Ango-dwaate gaa-izhisenig gii-gizhibizhigaadeni okaad, ogidigong onji.

Gii-ishkwaa-odaapinigaadenig okaad, gii-ayaa imaa ICU gaa-izhinikaadenig aakoziiwigamigong Jack. Aabiding dash imaa e-bimishing, ejakaabiigisijigaadegin onagizheyaabiinsan wenji-noondaagwaninig e-gii-gibichisenig ode' Jack. Daabishkoo awiya gii-ishkwaa-bimaadizid initaagwan.

Jack omaamaan imaa niibawiiban iwe gii-izhisenig. Odizhi-basiingweganaamaan ogozisan, "Ishe! Noojigo gidizhichige! Boonichigen gaa-izhichigeyin!" Aazha miinawaa obasiingweganaamaan. "Bimaadizin!" odinaan, "Gemaa giga-nishki'ish", odinaan.

Apane igi mashkikiiwininiwag gaye mashkikiiwikweg zhemaak onaajibatoonaawaa gaa-aabajitoowaad

Jack's leg wasn't healing. For six months now, the doctors had tried but the infection continued to eat his leg. In some areas, the flesh was completely gone, and you could see the naked bone that had been broken in the car accident. The pain was unbelievable.

"We're going to have to amputate," the doctor finally said. He was frank and kind all at once. Jack wasn't surprised and nodded his consent.

A week later his lower leg was gone, cut off below the knee.

After that amputation surgery, Jack spent a week in the hospital in the Intensive Care Unit. One day, the machine hooked up to his heart flatlined and sounded the continual beep of someone no longer alive.

Jack's mother was standing there beside the bed when it happened and she slapped him hard: "Stop fooling around, Jack," she shouted and slapped him again. "You better come back or I'm gonna be so mad at you!"

The doctors and nurses went running for the crash cart. Jack knew better than to disobey his mom, though. His heart ako awiya ode' gii-booni-anokiimaganinig. Jack dash o-gii-gikendaan ji-bizindawaad omaamaan. Gaa-izhi-maajii-anokiimaganinig miinawaa ode'. Aazha miinawaa bimaadizi gii-bagamibatoowaad mashkikiiwininiwag. Gaa-izhi-giiwebatoowaad iweni aabajichigan zhemaak.

Gaa-ishkwaa-giiged Jack bangii, o-gii-miinigoo' mashkikiiwininiwa' okaadikaan. Aaninda wendagidewan gaawiin dash aapiji onizhishinzinoonan. Giishpin dash wiin aakogindegin nawach onizhishinoon. Gaa-wendagidenig o-gii-ayaan. Gaawiin ako gii-minosinzinoon. Bezhigwek gegoon imaa gii-achigaadeni, amii dash ako ezhi-bakwajiseg iwe gaa-gii-izhiiginigaadeg. Ngoding ako gii-bimaakogoodeni okaadikaan Jack. Wiinge ko odagaji'igon gii-waabandang e-izhinaagwaninig iwe. Odazhiikewin gaa-izhi-dibendaagozid gaa-gii-diba'amowaad iweni. Amii dash gaa-izhi-giiwed, e-gii-maadanokiid miinawaa, e-wiiji-minikwemaadi' owiijiiwaagana'.

Gegaa ango-giizis e-izhisenig owiidoopamaan omaamaan Jack.

"Maamaa, wedi gii-ayaaying Montreal, gi-gii-nibaamin imaa nibewigamigong. Aapiji gii-onizhishin iwe nibewigamig,

machine was beating regularly again by the time the cart arrived, and the hospital staff turned right around, taking the crash cart with them.

After Jack had healed further, the doctors fitted him with an artificial leg, a prosthesis. Prostheses, though, are a little bit like cars. You can buy them cheaply made or you can buy them well made. Jack's new leg wasn't the best prosthesis. It rubbed at the stump. It didn't fit properly. It couldn't be locked into place – the whole thing was held in place by a single sheet of rubber at the stump so it would slip off too easily. Sometimes it would drag or slip out of place at a weird angle and people would look at Jack strangely. He would glance down then and see his leg, madly off in all directions. Kind of embarrassing. But it was the prosthesis that the Cree Board of Health paid for. He attached it to his stump as best he could and went back home. Back to work and to beers after work with the boys.

A few weeks later, Jack was having lunch with his mom.

"Mom, when we were in Montréal, we stayed in a hotel room. A really nice expensive room. With a big white bed and daabishkoo gaa-aakogindeg dinookaan. Gichi-nibewin, gaa-waabishkiigak gakina gegoon. Gii-baakiigaasinoon ini gaa-waabishkiigakin gibiiga'iganan. Gaa-waabishkaag gaye ishpimisag. Awiyag gii-gaagiigidowag agwajiing. Daabishkoo e-jiigakamigiziwaad imaa agwajiing. Aaniindi iwe? Aaniin dash gaa-onji-dediba'amang ji-ayaaying imaa?"

Oganawaabamaan ogozisan, awe ikwe. "Jack, gaawiin giin nibewigamigong gi-gii-ayaasii. Aakoziiwigamigong gi-gii-ayaa. Niin dash nibewigamigong. Gaawiin iwe gii-izhinaagwasinoon nibewigamig gaa-gii-izhi-nibaayaan."

"Ninganwiike iwe e-izhinaagwak," odinaan omaamaan, "Wiinge go nin-gikendaan imaa e-gii-ayaayaan."

"Gi-gii-nib. Gii-naagwan imaa biiwaabiko-makakong e-gii-niboyin. Gi-gii-bapasiingweganaamin dash, e-biibaagiminaan ji-bigiiweyin. Amii dash gaa-izhi-giiwe-bimaadiziyin. Wiinge gi-daa-gii-nishki'ish giishpin niboyamban."

Debwe dash iwe nibewigamig gii-ayaani gaa-gii-dazhindang. Gaawiin eta omaa akiing iwe gaa-ayaanig.

Gaa-ishkwaa-giizhitood gakina iwe gagwejiiwin gaa-gii-gikino'amawind ji-izhichiged ji-gashkitood ji-bimosed Jack, gii-giiwe e-wii-maadanokiid

white sheets and white curtains that blew in a bit with the breeze and a high white ceiling. People were talking outside the room. Like they were having a party in the hallway. Which hotel was that? How could we afford it?"

She looked at him a little strangely, and said, "Jack, you never stayed in a hotel. You stayed in the hospital and I stayed in a hotel. My hotel wasn't *anything* like that."

"But I remember," he said. "I'm sure of it."

"Boy, you died. That machine went into a flatline. I slapped you around a bit and yelled at you to come back. And it's a good thing you did, or I woulda been so mad at you."

That hotel room, it had been real, but it hadn't been in this world.

After Jack had finished all of the physiotherapy and recuperation stuff he was supposed to do, he got ready to head back to work. But just then, his boss miinawaa. Oganoonigoon odoogimaaman gii-dagoshing endaad. "Gaawiin ginandawenimigoosii ji-anokiiyin noopimiing miinawaa," odigoon odoogimaaman. "Aanawi gi-gashkitoon ji-babaamoseyin ji-aabajitooyin gikaadikaan, gaye apane go gi-nitaa-anokii. Giishpin dash gegoon izhiseyin noopimiing, ninaniizaanendaamin niinawind ji-bagamishkaagowaang giishpin gegoon izhiseyin," odigoon. "Omaa biindig gi-daa-gii-maadanokii, ozhibii'igewigamigong."

Gaawiin ozhibii'igewigamigong wii-anokiisii Jack. Wenjidoo go gaawiin.

Ogikendaan aapiji e-gii-gichi-gikino'amaazod. Gaye wiinge onagajitoon gete-bimaadiziwin bagwadakamig. Gaye gii-gikino'amawaa aaniin ge-ayizhiid noopimiing ji-anokiid, awensiwa' mitigoo' ji-naagaji'aad, gaye ji-aatawe'igewininiiwid. Ogashkitoon gaye niswayag ji-izhigiizhwed. Gaawiin daa-gwenawi-inanokiisii.

E-gii-wanitood dash okaad gaye odanokiiwin gii-onji-maanendam. Amii sa enaak e-inendang ji-goopaadenimidizod. Gii-maajii-minikwe. Gii-michi-nanaamadabi. Amii gaa-izhi-maajii-maanamanji'od, oziizibaakwadwaapinewin e-maanishkaagod. Aakoziiwigamigong ako ngoding gii-ayaa. Daga ndawaach

called him at home. The company didn't actually *want* Jack back at work as a conservation officer in the field, his boss said. With his new prosthesis, he was able to *do* the work, they could see that, and he had always been a good worker. But they were afraid of being sued if something went wrong for Jack and his artificial leg in the bush. They didn't want the liability. Instead, there was a desk job waiting that they thought would be perfect for him.

Jack didn't want to work at a desk. That was the end of that.

So far Jack had been an optimistic sort of guy. And he had quite a bit of education. He had studied traditional Cree ways on the land, he had studied to be a game warden and a wildlife conservation officer and a firefighter. He could speak three languages. He had options.

But losing a leg and a job in a matter of weeks was a bit much. He let go of his optimism and, for the first time in his life, he began to feel really sorry for himself. He did a whole lot of drinking and a whole lot of sitting around – which led to more diabetic and hypoglycemic comas and hospital stays. He even thought about killing himself and swallowed a bottle of

11

nin-daa-gii-nisidiz iinzan gii-maajii-
inendam. O-gii-gomaa' mashkikiwa'.
Gaawiin dash wiin debwe gii-wii-nibosii.
Wawaanendam aaniin ge-doodang. Aapiji
onandawenimaan awiyan ji-wiindamaagod
aaniin ge-izhichiged, noongom
e-gii-wanitood bezhig okaad gaye e-gii-
wanitood odanokiiwin.

Gaawiin dash awiyan ayaasiiwan
ge-gii-wiindamaagod ge-izhichiged.
Michi-minikwe. Michi-nanaamadabi.
Gwiiwizensan gaye gii-nitaawigiwan,
ogozisan. Gaawiin onandawenimaasiin
gii-bagijii nindede ji-inendamonid.

Ndawaach wiin eta ji-gikendang
ge-izhichiged.

Agaawaa gii-inendam ji-maajii-
naanaagadawendang aaniin
ge-gii-inanokiipan. Ganage abinoojiiyag
oshki-ayaag ji-wiiji'agwaa ndaa-inanokii
inendam. Maagizhaa ndaa-wiiji'aag
ji-nisidizosigwaa inendam. Giimooji-
wawiiyadendam wiin aaniish
gii-gagwe-nisidizooban gii-gomaad
mashkikiwa'. Maagizhaa ndaa-gashkitoon
ji-wiiji'agwaa inendam.

Okaad dash giiyaabi wiisagendam.
Giiyaabi miniiwanini. Gaawiin

pills. He didn't actually want to die, but
his life was turning out so differently from
what he had planned and expected. It was
confusing. He wanted all this sickness to
stop. He wanted comfort and attention. He
wanted someone to tell him it would be all
right. And it'd sure be nice to have someone
tell him what a guy like him was supposed to
do now, missing a leg and a job.

The problem was that there *was* no one,
really, who could tell him what to do or
who could change his situation. As long as
he was in a situation he didn't like, and as
long as he did nothing about it but drink
and sit around, he would continue to be
in the situation he didn't like. He had a
new son now too. He didn't want his kid to
think that his dad had given up.

He would have to figure it out for himself.

Begrudgingly at first, Jack pulled himself
together and started to think about
other ways he could make a living. He
had always wanted to work with kids. He
understood them. He had taken a course
in suicide prevention – funny for a guy
who had swallowed a bottle of pills – and
he knew some Cree kids were in trouble.
Maybe he had something to offer.

But that leg, the bad leg that had already
been amputated, was bothering him

ominoshkanziin iweni okaadikaan.
Ndawaach miinawaa Montreal gii-izhaa
ji-andawi'ind.

Gii-bimishin miinawaa aakoziiwigamigong
Jack. Aana-zaagidaabiigisinoon
onagizheyaabiinsan ji-zaagijijiwaninig
mini gaa-ozhi'oomaganinig wiiyawing.
Odaana-giziiyaabaawanaawaan gaye
e-zhizhoonamowaad boonzimigaanan.
Amii gaawiin. "Ndawaach miinawaa nin-
ga-odaapinaamin giiyaabi gikaad," odigoo'.
Imaa ishpiming inakeya'ii ogidigong
ji-izhi-giishkizhigaadenig okaad.

Wiinge noojigo wii-ikido epiichigidaazod.
Daa-gii-zhaaganaashiimo gemaa
daa-gii-baakwaa'ishiimo gaawiin dash
onandawenimaasii' mashkikiiwininiwa'
gaye mashkikiiwikwe' ji-noondaagod
noojigo ikidod. Ndawaach dash
gii-omashkiigoomo.

Miinawaa dash gii-maajizhwaaganiwi.
Nawach niibiwa okaad gii-odaapinigaadeni.

Odaanaang gii-maajizhond, gii-
nishkaadiziiban. Gaawiin dash
noogom wii-inendanzii iwe. Noongom
wii-wiiji'idizo. Amii gaa-inendang iwe
okaadikaan gaa-gii-miinind, odishkonigan

again. The prosthesis rubbed badly
against the stump. Sometimes the skin
rubbed right off and then it got infected
and he would have to go to Montréal for
infection control and it was all so familiar.

Wouldn't you know – Jack was in the
hospital being treated for infection
in the stump, and again they had the
drains carrying fluid out of the flesh, and
again they were washing the area with
antibiotics and applying treatments, and
again the treatments weren't working
and the flesh was being eaten away, and
again the doctor took a look. And said
they were going to have to amputate.
The same leg, up higher, above the knee.
Again.

Jack swore in Cree. He really wanted to
swear in English and French too, but he
didn't want the doctors and nurses there
to know he was swearing. So he just
swore some more in Cree and the others
in the room heard some words they had
probably never heard before.

A few days after that, he went into surgery
and woke up after. His leg stump now
ended in the middle of his thigh bone.

Last time, Jack had been eaten up with
anger and self-pity and it hadn't helped
at all. If he didn't want to go through the
whole stupid situation a third time, he
was going to have to help himself. The

gaa-gii-diba'amowaad, gaawiin onandawendaziin iwe. Ogikendaan gaawiin ji-ayaasig iwe. Nawach ji-agindenig onandawendaan. Bezhig ge-onizhishininig, weweni ji-gigishkang. Giishpin ngodwaak daswaak inagindeg iwe, maanoo inendam. Wiin gewiin o-da-diba'aan inendam.

Gaawiin ini zhooniyaan o-gii-ayaawaasiin. Zhooniyaawigamigong gii-izhaa e-gii-andooshkang ji-awi'ind iwe minik zhooniyaan. Debwe o-gii-debinaan. Gii-adaawe dash nawach gaa-agindenig okaadikaan. Zhiingendam. Zhaagooch dash o-gii-gashkitoon ji-debinang iwe. Amii gaa-izhi-giiwed gii-ishkwaa-achigaadenig iwe oshki-okaadikaan. Gii-giiwe. Anwebi imaa endaad, minikwe zhingobiiwaabo ji-na'imanji'od.

Iwe gii-ziizibaakwadwaapined, ngoding ako gii-nepidingwaamise, aakoziiwigamigong ako e-ayaad. Ngoding ako gaye jiita'odizo e-miinindizod iweni mashkiki gaa-inind ji-aabajitood. Amii dash ezhi-naanaagadawendang maagizhaa gaye ominikwewin gegoon gaa-inishkaagod. Gaawiin inendam. Aazha gegoon daa-gii-ikidowag mashkikiiwininiwag gaye mashkikiiwikwe.

prosthesis provided by the Cree Board of Health was not the prosthesis that Jack needed, he knew that now. His flesh infected so easily that he needed a much more expensive prosthesis, one that fit securely and could be locked into position and wouldn't rub off his skin. One that cost ten thousand dollars more than the prosthesis CBH provided. Jack would have to pay the difference himself.

Ten thousand dollars was a whole lot more money than Jack had. Either he had to come up with it or he had to get ready for the whole infection-amputation cycle to begin again. On crutches, Jack went to the bank, got a loan, and bought himself the expensive artificial leg. The situation was annoying – but at least he had been able to do something about it. After the new leg had been properly fitted, he went home, rested both legs on the coffee table and had a few beers to unwind.

Diabetic and hypoglycemic comas, and the inevitable hospital stays that came with them, were still a big part of Jack's life. Sometimes, as he injected himself with insulin, he wondered if his drinking had something to do with them, but surely, if that were the case, a doctor or nurse would have mentioned it somewhere along the way.

"Ngoding igo wiiba ndawaach gi-ga-giziiyaabaawanaag gidedikosiwag," odigoon mashkikiiwikwen. Gi-ga-izhaa na miinawaa Montreal?"

Gaawiin nakwetanzii Jack. O-michizhawiingetawaan. Odedikosiwa'? Ogikenimaa' awiya' gaa-giziiyaabaawanaawaad odedikosiwaa'. Giishpin iwe gewiin izhised gaawiin o-daa-gashkitoosiin bagwadakamig ji-izhaad. Aapiji onandawendaan ji-ando-gii'osed, ji-ando-gwaashkwebijiged. O-misawendaan imaa Iiyoo-ischiing ji-babaa-izhaad. Gaawiin onandawendaziin ji-giziiyaabaawanaad odedikosiwa'.

Apii gii-gashkitood gii-maajii-ayinaabi imaa maamaagoniganing, maagizhaa gegoon bakaan o-daa-gashkitoon ji-izhichiged. Debwe o-gii-mikaan. Bizaanigo daa-odaapiniganiwiwan odedikosiwan, bakaan dash odedikosiimaan daa-asaawan imaa. Bezhigwan gaye ini obiskwad daa-meshkwajimiinaa bezhig miinawaa. Amii ko netaa-igod mashkikiiwininiwa' gaawiin wiikaa daa-onji-mino-ayaasii gii-ziizibaakwadwaapined. Amii ji-nepiji-inaapined. Giishpin dash wiin oshki-obiskwad debinang, maagizhaa daa-onji-mino-ayaa inendam.

Miinawaa imaa gii-izhaad Montreal, o-gii-gagwejimaan mashkikiiwininiwan aaniin ezhisemagak gii-miinind oshkiya'ii imaa wiiyawing.

"You're going to need dialysis soon," a nurse said one day. "It's pretty clear that your kidneys are giving out. Will you be moving to Montréal, then, do you think?"

Jack smiled politely but didn't answer. His kidneys? He knew people on dialysis. Their lives were much more restricted than he wanted ever to be. He needed to be able to go to the bush. He needed to be able to hunt and fish. He needed to be able to move around Eeyou Istchee. Dialysis simply was not an option.

As soon as he was able, Jack began looking online for options other than dialysis. He found one – and it was every bit as drastic as amputation. He could have his kidney cut out and replaced with a transplanted kidney. He could also, at the same time, have his burnt-out pancreas replaced with a transplanted one. The doctors had always told him that there was no cure for diabetes. Once diabetic, always diabetic. But if he got a new pancreas, one not burnt out by diabetes, there was a chance that he might truly be cured.

At his next check-up in Montréal, Jack asked the doctor about transplanted organs.

15

"Gaawiin ganabach giin daa-minosesinoon iwe," odigoon mashkikiiwininiwan. "Ganabach daa-minose nawach ji-giziiyaabaawanadwaa gidedikosiwag. Niibiwa iwe izhichigewag."

O-michi-zhawiingwetawaan. Gii-apizo dash wedi gaa-izhichigewaad iwe mashkikiiwigamigong. Gii-gichi-gagwedwe. Ami dash gaa-igod ini mashkikiiwininiwa', giishpin wii-odaapinind iwe ji-izhitamawind, nawach babenak o-daa-doodaan oziizibaakwadwaapinewin. Daa-gagwe-mino-wiisini. Gaye daa-booni-minikwe. Giishpin iwe izhichiged, maagizhaa o-daa-wiiji'aawaan. Amii dash ge-izhi-bii'opan ji-inind bizaanigo ji-izhisepan iwe. Daa-asaa onaabiigamowining ji-bii'od baamaa awiyan ishkwaa-bimaadizinid bezhigewan dash omiskwiimiwaad daabishkoo, gaye dash gaa-inendang awe gaa-gii-nibod ji-aabaji'inind odedikosiwa'. Giishpin dash debinaad ini dedikosiwa' daa-miinaa mashkikiwa, gaye dash bizhishig daa-gagwejii gaye gaa-onizhishininig eta miijim ji-miijid gaye gaawiikaa ji-minikwesig gaye ji-aabajitoosig mashkiki gaa-jiikendamoshkaagemagak nepich igo. Gichi-naanaagadawendam. Maagizhaa gaye gaawiin o-daa-gashkitoosiin ji-miinind dedikosiwa'. Zhaagooch o-daa-gii-gojitoon. Aazha misawaach ozhiingendaan gii-nepidingwaamised ako, gaye gii-maanaakiziged.

"Oh Jack. I don't think you'd be a good candidate for that," the doctor said. "That's more a solution for – other people. But you could try dialysis. It's not so bad, you know. Lots of folks around here do it."

Jack smiled politely – then drove across town to the transplant clinic, where he asked question after question. Before transplant surgeons would even consider him for a transplant, the people at the clinic said, Jack would have to have his diabetes under better control and be regularly eating a healthy diet. Even harder, he would have to stop drinking altogether. If he managed to do those two things, then he might be eligible. If he was eligible, he'd be put on a list. After that, he would have to wait and see if anyone with healthy matching tissues died and donated her or his organs to people who needed them. If Jack got the organs, he would have to take special pills and he'd have to exercise and eat healthy and never drink alcohol and never get high for the rest of his life. It would be a big big deal and maybe in the end there would be no organs for him. But he could try. And he was getting pretty tired of comas and hangovers anyways. They had lost their appeal a long time ago.

Amii gaa-izhi-boonitood ominikwewin Jack. Gaye o-gii-boonitoonan ini gaa-jiikendamishkaagemagakin mashkikiwan. Gaawiin gii-izhaasii imaa gaa-izhaawaad gaa-booni-minikwewaad AA gaa-izhinikaadeg. Gaawiin misawaach imaa gii-ayaasinoon iwe dinookaan izhichigewin imaa Waswaanapiing iwe apii. Gaawiin awiyan ji-wiiji'igod. Amii gii-booni-wiijiiwaad owiijiiwaagana' gaa-zaagi'aapan. Ozaam giishpin gii-wiijiiwaad amii gaa-izhi-misawendang ji-minikwed. Amii gaa-izhi-nisidotang giishpin ginwesh wii-bimaadizid gaawiin memwaach ji-bekaabaawanaad odedikosiwa' zhaagooch igo ji-booni-minikwed gaye ji-booni-odaapinaad mashkikiwa'. Giishpin boonitoosig, gaawiin da-minosesii. Misawaach o-gii-ayaan bagwadakamig ji-izhaad. Giishpin gii-wii-minikwed, gii-ando-gwaashkwebijige ko, gemaa gii-ando-babaamibizo, gemaa gii-ando-babaamose noopimiing. Amii sa ginwesh amii gaa-izhichiged, e-gii-gwaashkwebijiged, ebabaamibizod, noopimiing e-babaa-ayaad. O-gii-minwendaan. Amii aaniish bizhishig gaa-gii-minwendang noopimiing gii-ayaad.

O-gii-gaganoonaan gaye ikwewan gaa-anokiinid imaa Waswaanapiing mashkikiiwigamigong. O-gii-waawiindamaagoon aaniin ge-gii-inanjiged, aaniin gaye enishkaagemagak iwe ziizibaakwadwaapinewin. O-gii-wiindamaagoon wegonen maawach

Jack quit drinking and he quit doing drugs. It was not easy at all. It was probably the hardest thing he had ever done. He attended no Alcoholics Anonymous nor Narcotics Anonymous group – Waswanipi had no such groups back then – and he had no support group. In fact, he had to stop hanging out with some of his closest friends for a while because, even though they were good people, when he was with them he wanted to drink. What he had was the knowledge that if he quit drinking and quit drugs, he stood a chance at a good life without dialysis; if he didn't quit, he had no chance at all. And he had the bush. Every time he wanted to drink, he went fishing, or for a drive, or out on the land. For a long time, it seemed that Jack spent most of his time fishing, driving, or out in the bush. That part wasn't so bad. The bush had always been his favourite place to be.

Jack began to speak with the new nutritionist who worked at the Waswanipi clinic. She explained to him what a healthy diet actually was and how diabetes works in the body, and she taught him ways to manage his diabetes with food. There were foods that made

ge-maanishkaagod daabishkoo
bakwezhigan, ziizibaakwad,
zhingobiiwaabo, gaye gegoonan
daabishkoo maakanoonii, gaye wegonen
wenizhishing daabishkoo bagwaji-wiiyaas
gaye gitigaanensan. Niibiwa gegoon
daa-gii-izhichige mewinzha giishpin
gikendangiban. Gaawiin dash o-gii-
gikendanziin. Gii-booni-minikwe. Gaye
bakaan gii-maajii-inanjige. Naano-giizis
gii-izhisenig gii-apizo wedi Montreal
imaa mashkikiiwigamigong gaa-izhi-
maajizhondwaa igi gaa-andawenimaawaad
oshki-dedikosiwa'.

O-gii-naanaagadawaabamaawaan weweni.
Gegoonan gaye o-gii-gagwejimaawaan.
Gii-meshkwadoonigaadeg gegoon
biinji-wiiyaw maawach zanagan. Giishpin
de-mashkawiziimaganzininig ode' gaawiin
daa-zhaabwiisii gii-maajizhond. Niibiwa
ayaawag awiyag gaa-andawendamowaad
ono dinookaanan. Giishpin dash Jack
gichi-inendanzig owe, giishpin maajii-
giiwe-minikwed apii minomanji'od,
gaye noojigo inanjiged, wiiba go
o-daa-maanzhi-doodawaa' ini gaa-gii-
miinind. Daa-miinaa aaniish mashkikiwa'
ji-onji-mino-ayaawaad ini dedikosiwa'.
Gaawiikaa daa-waniikesii ji-odaapinaad
ini mashkikiwa'. Ginwesh o-gii-
gaganoonaawaan. Apii gii-zaaga'ang imaa
mashkikiiwigamigong, amii gii-gashkitood
ji-asind imaa bii'onong, gewiin ji-bii'od
maagizhaa izhisenig awiyan ji-miinigod
dedikosiwan. Giishpin awiyan nibonid

it worse (breads, sugars, beer, pastas)
and foods that helped (traditional meats,
vegetables). In fact, he learned, there
were quite a few things he could have
done a long time ago to help manage
the disease. He just hadn't known about
them. Or if he had known, he hadn't taken
them seriously. Five months after his last
drink and after starting to eat differently,
he drove himself back down to the
transplant clinic in Montréal.

They looked him over carefully and asked
him questions. Organ transplant is one
of the most extreme surgeries that can
be done so they had to be sure that his
heart was strong enough to survive the
surgery. And there are more people
who need organs than who ever receive
them so they had to be sure that Jack
would respect the new organs. If he went
back to a life of drinking and of eating
in unhealthy ways, he would burn out
the organs very quickly. And anyone
who has had a transplant has to take
pills to convince the immune system to
accept the new organs. Those pills can't
be forgotten even once. Their list of
questions and tests was long and intense.
But, by the time Jack left the clinic, he
was on a list for new organs. If someone
with healthy organs and matching tissues
died, he could receive their organs.

bezhigwan dash izhi-omiskwiimiwaad,
daa-miinaa ini dedikosiwan.

Nitam dash gii-izhi'aa
ji-giziiyaabaawanaad odedikosiwa'.
Gaawiin gii-anokiisiiwa' odedikosiwa
ji-zaagijisemagak gaa-maanaadak
gegoon wiiyawing. Daa-bekaagaminini
omiskwiim giishpin wii-debinaad oshki-
dedikosiwa'. Endaso-niizho-giizis Montreal
gii-izhaa nising endaso-dwaate, e-gii-
namadabid imaa e-giziiyaabaawazonid
odedikosiwa'. Niibiwa omashkiigoo'
imaa o-gii-waabamaa'. Gii-jiikendamoo'
awiyan e-ayaanid ge-gaganoonaawaad.
Gii-jiikendam gewiin Jack.

Aabiding dash gii-noondam awiyan iinzan
ozaam wiiba gii-nibowan, o-daa-debinaan
dash ini dedikosiwan. Gii-aakozi dash iwe
gaa-giizhigak Jack. Gaawiin dash o-gii-
gashkitoosiin ji-debinaad ini dedikosiwan.
Awiya bakaan gii-maajizhwaa e-gii-
miinind ini dedikosiwan. Miinawaa
dash ningoding igo, Waswaanipiing
wii-izhaaban Jack. Gii-wiindamawaa
awiyan miinawaa e-gii-nibonid. Gii-ayaa
ndawaach imaa Montreal Jack e-bii'od.
Debwe dash gii-miinaa iwe apii 2012
gii-izhisenig oshki-dedikosiwan gaye
obiskwad.

Jack eta bezhigo omaa mazina'iganing
e-gii-ayaad ziizibaakwadwaapinewin
gaawiin dash noongom. E-ayaad oshki-
obiskwad, gaye e-gashkitoomaganinig

In the meantime, the doctors put him on
temporary dialysis. His own kidneys could
no longer flush out all the toxins they
were supposed to flush out, but his blood
had to be free of toxins if he was to live
through such a rigorous surgery. For two
months, he went into the Montréal dialysis
clinic three times a week and sat there
for four hours as the big dialysis machine
cleaned his blood. Again, he met many
Cree people there who needed someone
to talk to and Jack was happy to oblige.

One day, he heard that someone had
died too soon and organs had become
available for him. But for some reason
Jack had a fever that day and his surgery
had to be cancelled. The organs went
to someone else on the list. Not too
long after that, Jack was about to catch
a plane to Waswanipi for a visit when
someone else died too soon. Jack stayed
in Montréal and, on that day in 2012,
he received a new kidney and a new
pancreas.

Jack is the one person in this book
who once had diabetes but no longer
does. Because he has a new pancreas,
and because his body accepts the

owiiyaw ji-aabajitoomaganinig ziizibaakwadwaapine-mashkiki insulin gaa-izhinikaadeg, wiinge noongom mino-ayaa Jack. Wiinge go mino-ayaa. Noongom dash aapiji onaagadawaabandaan wegonen gaa-miijid. Gaawiin omiijisiin gaa-adaawaadenig wiisiniiwigamigoonsing wewiib gaa-ayaamagak. Wiin igo ogiizizaan ge-miijid. Wiiyaas gaye gitigaanensan omiijinan gaawiin dash aapiji maakanoonii gaye opiniin. Gaawiin gaye minikwesii gaye ji-odaapinang mashkiki gaa-jiikendamoshkaagemagak. Moozhak noopimiing ayaa, amii aaniish imaa ezhi-minwendang ji-ayaad. O-gikino'amawaan ogozisan bizaanigo bagwadakamig ji-ondaadizinid, bizaanigo e-ayaad okaadikaan gaye oshki-odedikosiwa' gaye oshki-obiskwad giiyaabi mino-bimaadizi. Andomoozwe, obigiiwewidoon ako moonzowiiyaas gaye godag dinookaan wiiyaas. Giizizekwe. Gagwejii. Ngoding ako dewaawigane gii-ayekozid ozaam okaadikaan e-ayaad. Onizhishinini dash gii-gagwejiid, gaye noopimiing gii-babaa-ayaad. Giishpin gii-ojaanimendami'igod gegoon gichi-ayaan ogaganoonaan. Gaye gaa-inanokiinid iwe ogaganoonaan.

Ngoding ako onaanaagadawendaan giiwanimowin. Giishpin awiya gwayak gaganoonigopan gii-oshkaadizid maagizhaa bakaan

insulin it creates, he is actually cured of the disease. His new pancreas works beautifully, and his new kidney feels fine. But transplanted organs have to be handled very carefully. Even though he no longer has diabetes, he is more vigilant about health than he ever was before. He avoids fast food, he cooks his own meals (mostly meat and vegetables with a little bit of pasta or potatoes), and he doesn't drink or do drugs even a little bit. Since the bush is where he has always felt healthiest, he spends as much time on the land as he can. He teaches his son the traditional ways of the land so that his son knows that even a robot leg and transplanted organs can't stop you from living on the land if it's what you want to do. He hunts and brings home moose and other game, and he cooks it up. He exercises when he can. His lower back often aches from the extra work it has to do with an artificial leg and his flesh-and-blood foot sometimes gets swollen from all the exercise, but exercise is what has to happen if he wants to stay healthy, and so Jack does it. When he's stressed out about life in general, he talks with an elder, and when he's stressed out about work, he talks to a psychologist so the stress doesn't bottle up inside.

Sometimes he thinks about bullshit. He heard piles of it over the years. Maybe if someone had been direct with him when he was younger, his diabetes would not

daa-gii-izhi-bimaadizi, gaawiin dash
daa-gii-izhi-gichi-ziizibaakwadwaapinesii.
Giiyaabi o-daa-gii-ayaan okaad
gaye odedikosiwan gaye obiskwad.
Ngoding giiyaabi onoondaan
giiwanimowin. Aabiding o-gii-igoon gaa-
maamiinomiwenid gaawiin ji-izhaasig
noopimiing e-nabanegaaded. Gaawiin
gegoon gii-ikidosii Jack. Apane gii-gii'ose.

O-gii-gagwejimigoon awiyan noongomiike
giishpin e-inendang daabishkoo e-oshki-
maajitaad oshki-dedikosiwan e-ayaawaad.

"Daabishkoo e-gii-miinigoo'aan gegoon
nindinendaan," ikido, "ambegish dash eta
nawach wiiba owe izhisegiban."

Gaawiin onishki'igosii'
mashkikiiwininiwa' gaa-gii-
mamaanzhiinid. Gaawiin awiyan
wii-dibaakonaasiin. O-gii-wiindamawaan
bezhig owiijiiwaaganan giishpin
dibaakonaapan ini mashkikiiwininiwan
apii gii-gizhibizhigaadenig okaad, daa-
gi-gichi-ozhooniyaami. Maagizhaa dash
gaye o-daa-gii-michi-minikwaanaan
ozhooniyaaman. Aanjiike dash
daa-gii-maanzhiiyaa. Gaawiin gaye
o-nishki'igosiin odoogimaaman
gaa-gii-webaakonigod. Gaawiin gaye
onishki'igosii' ini gaa-wendagidenig
okaadikaan gaa-gii-miinigod.
Nawach o-gichi-inendaan weweni

have become so severe and he might
still have his original leg and kidney and
pancreas. Sometimes he still runs into
bullshit. A counsellor told him not long
ago that he had to accept that his time
in the bush was over, that hunting was
not something a one-legged man should
do. Jack smiled politely – then left the
clinic to go hunting. The way to deal with
bullshit is to help yourself.

Not long ago, someone asked him if he
felt like his new organs had given him a
second chance. He thought about it for a
while.

"Not a second chance, exactly," he said.
"I feel like the Lord came through. But a
little too late."

He's not angry at the doctors who made
so many mistakes, and he doesn't want
to sue anyone for malpractice. He told
a friend once that, if he had sued back
when his leg had to be amputated
because of a doctor's mistake, he would
just have had more money, which he
would have spent on more drinking and
partying, which would have led to even
more health problems. Nor is he angry at
his bosses who didn't want the liability of
having him working in forestry. He's not
even angry at the people who provided a
cheap prosthesis that only irritated his leg
further and led to a second amputation.
What he wants is to move on, to continue

noongom ji-bimaadizid, ji-minochiged obimaadiziwin.

Anokii dash e-maamiinomaad oshkaadizii' imaa Waswaanipiing, gaye owiijitoon iwe izhichigewin gaa-izhi-maamowiinowaad anishinaabeg gaye eshkiimeg imaa Kwebec gaye Labrador. Gaye oniigaanishkaan ji-boonichigaadeg nisidizowin. Gaye owiidanokiimaa' omashkiigoo' ji-wiiji'indwaa awiyag gaa-ositaawisewaad giishpin gashkitoosigwaa ji-bimosewaad daabishkoo gaa-maakiziwaad. Wiin gaye owiiwan onaagaji'aawaa' abinoojiizha gaa-ayaawaasinind oniigi'igowaa'. Apane o-wiiji'aa ji-ganoonind aaniin igo apii.

Ini oshkaadizii' gaa-wiidanokiimaad gewiinawaa niibiwa noojigo gegoon onoondaanaawaa. Amii dash enaad ako, "Giishpin gwayak izhi-bimaadizisiyeg amii gegiinawaa owe ge-izhiseyeg gaa-gii-izhiseyaan." Owiindamawaa' weweni ji-naagaji'idizonid, ji-booni-minikwenid gaye gaa-onizhishing miijim ji-miijinid gaye ji-booni-miigaadinid, wegonen igo ji-onji-mino-bimaadizinid. Debwewin eta owiindamawaa', wiinawaa eta o-daa-gashkitoonaawaa ji-wiiji'idizowaad, ji-mino-bimaadiziwaad. Gii-ikidod ako iwe, owaabandaanaawaa e-nabanegaadenid amii dash ezhi-debwetawaawaad.

Giiyaabi dash omikwenimaa' ini omashkiigoo'

to live the good life he has, to contribute in meaningful ways.

He works as a counsellor and suicide prevention officer with the youth of Waswanipi, is on the Board of Directors for First Nations and Inuit of Québec and Labrador, and is the co-president of Suicide Prevention in the region. He also works with the Cree Board of Health to protect the livelihoods of people with disabilities, he and his wife foster kids and provide a safe home for them when they can't be with their parents, and he is on call with Youth Protection.

The youth he works with have heard piles of bullshit too. So he tells them direct, straight off the bat, "Look, this is what you gotta do. If you don't do it, this is what will happen." He tells them to look after themselves, or to stop drinking, or to eat healthier, or to stop fighting, or to do whatever they can do to improve their situation. He tells them the truth, all of it, including how they can help themselves, including that it's up to them to make their own lives better. When he says that, they look at his robot leg and believe him.

He still thinks of all the Cree who suffer alone in the hospitals. Eventually, after his